About the book

Title: 3 hours sex

Five evils that hang over the well-being and sexual health of modern man: Diabetes, hypertension, stress, impotence and premature ejaculation.

Over 80% of the male population, for various reasons, suffer or will suffer from sexual impotence and premature ejaculation.

Are you wanting to be part of that statistic?

In this ebook, you will find ways to prevent, eliminate or drastically alleviate this prediction.

And the best of cheap, healthy and efficient manner; without ingesting expensive drugs and harmful side-effect its Saide and longevity.

That's right: it's mis since White Magic helping you.

Fifteen types of spells to make you feel refreshed and invigorated to have sex with ever imagined in your life.

Problems? contact us at the website below:

http://www.topbook.com.br

We guarantee absolute discretion and confidentiality.

ATTENTION: it is recommended to consult a cardiologist before beginning the following advice and recommendations of this eBook, and especially the spells, because they are strong.

Preface

With this ebook, you will become the favorite subject of the female audience; the unforgettable good lover.

Second only to sexual impotence, premature ejaculation is the largest ghost, for that matter, a major cause of mismatch between sexual partners. It is the natural and inexorable order of nature, to have healthy and profitable act erection is necessary; to meet the woman or passive partner, it is necessary to eliminate the erection and premature ejaculation remain, that which occurs in less than 40 minutes.

Premature ejaculation, and the consequent full partner of the non-satisfaction still leads to man various other problems such as:

- Low self esteem;

- Betrayal Risk

- Sex Trail;

- Stress;

- Depression;

- Embarrassment;

- Insecurity;

- Social Misfit;

- Segregation.

Prevent yourself. get rid of this problem that affects a large range of the male population.

In this ebook, you'll have everything for this: lasting erections and ejaculations supercontroladas to meet the most demanding woman in the world.

See the link below to get enthroned materials at Mage Sidrak

http://topbook.com.br/consecrated-hexagram#Hexagram

Advices

"If advices was good, no one gave, sold".

By agreeing with this intelligent and real thesis, we wrote this Ebok, which is not free, like other materials, superficial and biased that are seen around blurred realism and without any productive practical result.

When we talk about prolonged sex means more partners fucking hours, not counting in that time, with brief

interruptions for affection, conversation, hydration and food and, of course, preliminary as dinner and dancing.

Ignore orgasm means continuing the relationship, even after cum - logical that for this it is necessary to be able to maintain an erection, or rather minimize the response time to new erection - which does not exceed, so you're knowledge of all content ebook ten minutes negligible.

The man, active, want to minimize, always ejaculation, while women, or passive partners, are free to enjoy all they want.

For being obvious and commonplace, although very important, not We mention, in any tips chances of physical exercise.

Various suggestions, advice, are directed to men (active part) because there is no woman in the world, even women who are not ready for more than three hours of unrestricted and uninterrupted sex.

Doubt? Ask your partner, or any other woman you have that freedom.

So let's get down to business:

Conditioning

• Do not ejaculate for 2 or 3 days

Every time you ejaculate, your body spends energy to replenish the liquid, which is actually a complex substance of nutrients - carbohydrates, minerals, proteins, vitamins, lipids, water - lowering the quality of the next erection by increasing the time recovery and decreasing libido. Even though relationship, stay for 3 days without enjoying even though the control at the beginning is difficult. Make your ejaculation an act of pleasure, not a necessity.

• Relax

For you not to give in to the impulse to enjoy, relax, think about other things than sex. For 20 minutes, be silent, alone - can be while she bathes - thinking in nature, in birdsong, etc. This will relieve the stress and the expectation of sex.

• Detach the brain's bed

Only one way of something never-ending: there is a beginning. Make love and caresses a routine. Unbind the pleasure of the place, that is, the act of enjoying tied to the bed. Indulge in all that is around you: mentally make love with wine, furniture, seats. In this way, you begin to penetrate the woman, her mind will imagine that you are much longer in it, so come to orgasm more quickly - you watching everything cabin without cease affection - while maintaining the erection.

• Do not force never

We have no obligation to end a perfect evening with sex. If you are tired, nervous, have drunk too much, better not start anything. Rest, Sleep; tomorrow is a new day. This is preferable to doing a casual sex without force, apathetic. If the partner is lively, you should take a cold shower - temperature below 24 degrees Celsius. If, even then, will not come naturally, forget, or let the woman get excited and ask for penetration. The point is not settle for a vigorous sex, careful, with full dedication both.

• Breathe properly

To have sex, you spend energy. Energy at the cellular level, is achieved in a reaction that consumes water, oxygen and glucose.

So learn to breathe correctly: most women They make the lung, shallow breathing, even during sex; man, even to do that in normal activities, can not afford to breathe this way during the act. Man should breathe through abdomen. The usual belly contraction should be transferred to the pelvic muscles. That's the correct way to breathe, never using the excess diaphragm.

PRACTICE!

Soon as this fact becomes reflex.

• Constant erection

Is an accomplice of his partner, accomplice-lover. If today we enjoy easily, because it is not yet understand the game. Otherwise, not exchange hours of revitalizing pleasure for hours sleepy tiredness. We would do everything to prevent orgasm end the game. Well, to recognize a game, invent and simulate him to realize that he was always there. Talk to your partner so that it, when you're having sex, you do not stop until you are ready to sleep. She makes use of hands, breasts, lips and feet to sustain his erection in the intervals between penetration and another. The idea is to fall into apathy for a minute.

• Lubricant

Long hours of sexual practice, requires lubrication. Natural does not always support this marathon, especially in women after fifty years. Leave this product within reach of his hand.

• breaks

Take breaks during the pleasure of practice time. Every hour, take a breath, drink water generously and eat some sort of fruit, peanuts, nuts.

• Every man is sexually impotent at times

Do not worry if this happens from time to time. Even once a month, according to experts, it is normal. However, if you feel uncomfortable, seek proper medical guidance. The best way to redeem a paperback is not to give much importance to it.

In such cases paperback, give up trying to accept defeat and smiled. If you do not, then yes fall in hopeless classic paperback. If, instead, laugh and let go all of a sudden your hands will be walking on her body and the whole situation will arise again.

• Donate up, focus on your partner

It is very common to find women and men to enjoy, focus on their own feelings and to turn a blind eye, cloistered, contracted, as teenagers in their first orgasms. To avoid that sex becomes a masturbation to two, the path is the reverse. When getting lost within yourself, point your gaze to the other, offer your pleasure, dip, drop, scratch your man, stick, earth, goal harder on his wife. Only when we are distracted we enjoy watching our feelings.

• Medications

Some medicines for certain illnesses such as depression or various psychological disorders, affect the quality of erections, so that is recommended before starting any prolonged treatment, consult your specialist about its effects on your sex life. Also the excesses of alcohol, tobacco and drugs affect your health and also your erections, keep this in mind and control yourself.

• Free yourself

Make use of sex toys and fantasies, with mutual consent of the partners. These are not just to have fun with your partner or try new things, but they can also help increase your power. The penis rings were expressly designed to improve erection, have a very simple to use and which undoubtedly will make their sexual relationships are much more intense, vigorous and enjoyable.

* Although this matter at first glance, seems exclusively directed to heterosexual men, we made it clear that we have nothing against homo-affective relations.

Foods

You are what you eat!

This is one of the wisest sayings that exist. We, living beings are made up of chemicals in dosing and appropriate percentage for our birth, growth, strengthening and maintenance of healthy living. If these concentrations change significantly, our body will react adversely to our claims, focusing on a variety types of deficiencies and problems that we carry for the rest of our lives. In sex life, this is no different.

To enhance your sexual performance, in quality and quantity, go to consume the suggested foods:

• Zinc

Increase intake of zinc, since this mineral plays a role important in testosterone production that influences the desire and sexual performance.

Folic acid and zinc are essential to maintain the quality of

sperm. Without folic acid, reduces the number of sperm and their movement is weak. And without zinc, growth and development of sex organs are affected negatively. Folic acid is found in foods rich in vitamin B6. The chicken is one of the foods with folic acid and zinc, which help to improve sperm quality. Pumpkin seeds and oysters are other important sources of zinc, very beneficial for sperm.

• Carbohydrates and proteins

Consume a good amount of carbohydrates and protein to maintain a good level of energy that will allow you to have more and better sexual activity.

• Salt

Drastically decrease your salt intake.

• Fatty Food and processed

Abandon, or at least greatly decreases the consumption of canned foods, sausages and other foods high in fat. When preparing meat, remove, before cooking, the majority of visible fat.

• Increase your intake of white meat, fish, vegetables, fruit.

• If you are not hyperuricaemic or hipercolesterêmico (high cholesterol) (high uric acid), in short, under dietary restriction, consume fruit-fish once a week.

• Vitamins

Vitamins act as catalysts in our body. Fat-soluble vitamins can be stored (fat-soluble), as water-soluble vitamins (dissolved in water) did not. Vitamin C is essential for improving the quality of sperm production, since their antioxidant properties stimulate the movement of sperm. Orange, lemon and kiwi are excellent sources of this vitamin. It is recommended to drink at least a glass of orange juice a day to improve sexual performance. There are other sources of this vitamin.

Vitamin E is another powerful antioxidant essential for the improvement of sperm and can be found mainly in vegetable oils and dried fruits. However, foods rich in vitamin E, more effective for improving sperm quality are walnuts, almonds, wheat germ and olive oil.

Vitamin A influences the formation of androgen steroids, Essential for the creation of sex cells and therefore favors the quality of semen and fertility. Foods rich in vitamin A that benefit most from the improvement of sperm are dairy products, carrots, pumpkin and spinach.

• Fatty acids

Omega 3 and omega 6 are essential for improving sperm, since the fatty acid and linolenic acid are essential for proper maturation process of spermatozoa. The main foods rich in these substances that improve the quality of sperm are nuts, flaxseed and fish.

• Garlic

Garlic is a food that favors considerably sperm production, improved heart function, reduces blood sugar and cholesterol, among many other benefits.

Surprisingly, other foods which improves the quality of Sperm is popcorn, since it has a high level of plant arginine, which is a major component of the sperm.

• Infusions

Mint is one of the first medicinal plants used in aphrodisiac purposes, so your tea is considered one of the best to activate sexual desire and increase libido. If this ingredient alone, is a potent natural aphrodisiac, if you add another major nervous system stimulants, such as cinnamon, the result is an impregnated infusion of flavors and flavor able to awaken **its most hidden instincts.**

The cardamom tea is an excellent natural aphrodisiac because of its high content of zinc, an essential mineral for the stimulation of sex cells. This plant, originally from India, is highly beneficial to improve blood circulation and regulate the digestive system. To enhance its aphrodisiac properties and best results, a perfect option is to add to this brew a tablespoon of ground coffee, because it is another natural stimulant of the nervous system.

The vanilla beans have a potent euphoric power, which allows combat sexual apathy and increase the libido levels.

Since ancient times, Indians use this natural product for flavoring environments, providing a relaxing atmosphere and encourage passion for sexual encounters. Its relaxing properties, aroma and flavor make it one of the most aphrodisiac infusions and natural stimulants sexual desire.

Many cultures consider the ginger one of the largest natural aphrodisiacs for men. Thanks to its powerful stimulating effect the nervous system, allows more strong and durable erections. To increase their aphrodisiac properties, we can combine it with a little honey because honey is also considered stimulating sexual desire due to minerals that compose it.

Finally, ginseng stands out as one of the infusions

aphrodisiac. This is because it has the ability both to improve male erections as to increase libido in women. However, it is important to highlight their intake conditions as ginseng, although it has many benefits, it also presents a number of contraindications we should consider.

Heads up:

As with all medicinal plants, we must take special care to take them and consider both the benefits and the contraindications. Therefore, it is not advisable to ingest more than two cups daily aphrodisiac infusions or take them every day for a long period of time. We are advised to always carry out every three to five days and consult with a specialist about which infusions can be switched and which can not, in your particular case.

As for the best time to eat them, experts recommend not to do immediately after a meal, wait at least an hour for this.

Secrets

The sexual position chosen can also influence the erection quality. Those that is above or vertically as the "four", the mission, trapezium or deep allow blood to flow better, helping to maintain an erection for a longer time, which does not occur as effectively when itIt is over. This does not mean that one should never play other positions, but to take into account if your goal is to last a little longer than usual.

One of the most common reasons why men have trouble controlling the ejaculatory reflex is inadequate masturbation.

Although it seems an easy task, not all realize it so correct, triggering premature ejaculation during sex.

Therefore, one way to avoid this is to masturbate properly. If you normally do it quickly, to satisfy his excitement as soon as possible, your body becomes used to produce quick orgasms, a fact that will be seen reflected at the time of having sex.

If your case, what should you do to prevent premature ejaculation is to try to control the masturbation so that orgasm occurs later. The best way to do it is to press with the thumb and index finger the part that is under the glans, when you feel the need to ejaculate; when decreasing continue with masturbation. Do not forget to enjoy the moment and relax.

And your mood?

If during the sexual encounter anything that worries you, if you suffer from a stress or anxiety framework for whatever reason or feel bored, most likely the relationship will not be the desired and end in premature ejaculation. To prevent that from occurring, you should spend a few minutes a day to perform relaxation techniques which enable it to shut down what worries during their sexual relationships and focus only on their own pleasure and partner.

Besides controlling masturbation and perform relaxation techniques, there are other exercises to avoid premature ejaculation very effective. Among them, there is the Kegel technique, which is to stop the flow of urine for a few seconds and expel it in small quantities, once relaxed.

In case you have a partner, treat sexual disorders is something of both. So if your premature ejaculation is not sporadic, and if it is a common problem during the first few months, performing the exercises to avoid it and masturbation techniques, it is advisable to note, too, the sexual positions that you practice . Opt positions as spoon or jellyfish, characterized by not allowing the penis to penetrate through and reach orgasm later, thereby preventing premature ejaculation.

Performing a process of cleansing and detoxifying the body is very important to prevent the accumulation of toxins, which also affect the control of the ejaculatory reflex. In this regard, the juices are very effective antioxidants.

Spells

"Of doctor, sorcerer and crazy all have a little."

Let touch on your connection with the supernatural and enjoy yourself of privileges.

Whenever you feel exhausted or decreased in your sexual stamina, do one of these rituals, or all of them (never both).

1 - Basil materials

1 kit of magic with towel and athame, enthroned

21 basil leaves;

5 liters of filtered water;

White clothes to sleep.

Preparation

Place the towel with the pentagram on top of a table, with athame on the right side;

Load materials above on the towel;

Place the basil leaves in the container with 5 liters of water;

On low heat, let the water heat, without boiling, and remove from heat.

Application

Before bed, take your usual bath;

Wipe up with a clean, white or blue color;

Carefully soak up, from the neck down, with prepared above;

Wait until the drain liquid and evaporates naturally;

Dress for sleeping with white clothes;

Do this ritual for 21 days, consecutive.

Keep zealously the towel and the athame.

2 - Corn cob

Materials

01 ear of corn beautiful, long, thick and lush

01 very strong cock

01 papaya-female and mature

01 athame, enthroned

01 Red spool of thread

01 needle

Preparation:

Before sunrise, the last day of full moon, threshing corn, with the aid of athame;

Book seven grains and give all the rest to the cock eat;

Do with the athame, a hole in the papaya without pierce papaya, to fit the ear;

Thread the cob of corn inside the papaya, leaving the cable

cob out;

Remove the quick and, through the hole, remove seven papaya seeds;

Place the seeds in red velvet bag;

Close this bag, using the thread and needle;

One should not give us the line or cast off at the end;

Return the cob into the papaya and bury them in the root of a tree;

Without your partner know it, put the bag under the couple's mattress.

• This ritual should be fully completed before by sunsets.

 3 - Avocado Pit

materials

01 avocado pit

01 black or blue felt tip pen

01 athame

01 good quality brandy bottle

Preparation:

Take an avocado seed and let it dry in the sun for 3 days;

Then write your name in stone, with a felt-tip pen, and cut the core into small pieces, patiently with the athame;

Put the pieces into the bottle of brandy and bury it in a flower garden, saying:

"Forest beings, receive this offering as proof of my respect for you. In return, I ask that increase my sex drive!"

Then go away without looking back.

 4 - Clothing

material

1 underwear

1 hexagram enthroned

Preparation

Buy a underwear - the best you have conditions financial to acquire;

One evening crescent, use it for the first time, with the hexagram to the neck;

Sleep with her;

On the morning of the next day, place it at the highest point of a

banana;

Use the hexagram the neck, always;

Browse never go through these site.

5 - Perfume

The lack of sexual vigor is something that can destroy the married life. But sometimes the problem may be linked to negative energies that hinder the time to satisfy his partner.

Proceed as follows:

Grab some Orange perfume, you find in perfume houses;

The mattress where the couple sleeps, skip the perfume shaped cross, the 4 corners of the mattress;

Do not tell your partner about it.

Program that special night and see what happens.

When the aroma starts to wear off, re sympathy.

6 - Gems

2 chicken eggs D'Angola

1 cup enthroned

preparation

Prepare an eggnog with eggs;

Put it in the cup and stir in the honey;

Take a sip before intercourse.

Your mate will delirious, especially if both drink this "elixir".

7 - Esoteric bath

1 kit enthroned spells

1 Sword of St George into strips, cut with athame

20 liters of clean water

Incense: musk

6 purple candles

1 mug

Preparation bath

The bath should be prepared by boiling up the sword strips;

Let stand for 15 min;

Strain;

It's ready!

Take care bath;

Light the incense near you;

Light the candles;

Then throw the contents of esoteric bath, head down - play slowly with the aid of mug;

Herbs and other materials used in the bath and smoking should be dispatched later in tap water.

Save the kit and the remaining instruments.

8 - Patois

Get some water lily flowers.

Take a piece of orange cloth.

Wrap the water lily flowers in this piece of cloth and sew it with the orange line.

This is a strong patuá to improve sexual appetite.

Never leave without taking it in the bag or even stuck on the inside of your clothing.

9 - Tape

This sympathy should be made by the wife on the day of the month with the number seven. Example: 7, 17, 27.

Take 30 cm white tape, any width;

Write to the fullest extent of the tape the name of your husband.

Then tie this tape a picture of your husband, placing it in a church, at the foot of the saint you to be devout;

Pray, soon after three Save Queens.

10 - Keep fervent partner

1 red towel;

1 vase with ***me-anyone-can**

Procedure

Has relations with him;

Then wipe it with a towel;

Bury it in the pot;

When the ***plant** is very pretty, let her near a tree

leafy, always visualizing you and him, or to have it in your home, but never forget to take care of it.

11 - To increase sexual stamina and eliminate frigidity

Fill a bottle with filtered water;

Scroll to a crib - a church - and ask Jesus to bless the water, so it can heal, relieve, finally, carry all evil and bring all good;

Use this water year round and ask for what you want or need, for example, play in the corners of your home and ask what is right and take the issue far away;

You can also drink, in short, has all utilities and power.

12 - "*Garrafada*"

The gypsy garrafada is famous for its quick results.

Proceed as indicated that the effects will be amazing.

materials

1 liter of dry white wine;

1 cup enthroned

1 kit spells, enthroned

Cloves;

ginger;

Bread crumb;

1 apple;

Cinnamon in Pau;

1 Galician Lemon;

1 piece of lettuce from the ground;

Pata 1 egg;

1 pinch of salt;

3 Green Grapes;

1 piece of Marmalade.

Preparation

Put everything in a bowl and mix;

Divide into bottles and cap well;

Leave for three days in a cool place.

Dosage

Drink a cup three times a day.

13 - "domestic Viagra"

ingredients

1 liter of pure watermelon juice

1 large lemon, if small, is used-two

1 cup enthroned

1 kit enthroned spells

1 knife

preparation

Arrange watermelon in sufficient quantities for one liter of juice, the pulp removed, use a knife to cut the watermelon;

With the athame, cut into pieces the flesh;

Extract the juice with juicer, a blender or whisk;

Strain and transfer the juice to a saucepan;

Bring to a boil for about 4 minutes;

Squeeze a large lemon without the seeds directly on the boiling juice;

Mix well, and let it continue boiling until the liquid is reduced by half;

Turn off the heat and allow to cool for about an hour;

Meanwhile, prepare a glass bottle which can be closed tightly;

Pass the aphrodisiac potion for the bottle, and store it in the refrigerator.

How and when to drink?

Always drink on an empty stomach, preferably fasting in 40 ml doses per day, using the cup;

Even after feeling good, never ceases to drink it at least every other day.

This cup can only be used by you.

NOTE

The following white magic are not recommended for heart disease, people who have suffered strokes and men over sixty years, unless there is express medical release.

14 - Glass

ingredients

01 drink dose cup

01 cup enthroned

01 kit spells, enthroned

01 hexagram enthroned

01 American Cup

01 Lemon socador

01 clove garlic, minced

01 tablespoon chopped onion coffee

01 teaspoon ground cinnamon coffee

1/4 minced chilli pepper

01 coffee spoon

01 good quality condom

01 elastic

01 knife

01 bay leaf chopped

1 table

1 liter of dry red wine

Preparation

One night Crescent Moon, may be the first or second night, put the ingredients on the table, having the kit on it;

Place the hexagram in the neck;

In the American glass, add the chopped garlic, loro, minced onion, cinnamon and pepper;

With the help of juicer (pestle) and punch it all until a homogeneous mixture (about five minutes);

If lock-in some lonely place in your home and masturbate;

Play the expelled semen in the dose cup;

Pour the contents of the American cup, all have macerated in that

dose cup (use a teaspoon to assist);

Very slowly and calm, mix it all;

With condoms, make a seal that glass, mouth to the bottom;

Place the elastic catching and tying it all.

Order and prayer

The next day, before dawn the sun, take this cup prepared and head to a large tree, the best you can find;

With the help of athame, make a hole in the ground with about seven centimeters;

Bury the glass that hole, covering the earth;

Recite softly, with great faith and concentration, looking for that hole plugged, the following prayer three times:

Note: take the prayer printed on a piece of paper to read at the appropriate time.

"I invoke the Lord of all things, creator of the universe and everything in it. I invoke the God who created Salomon, King's favorite, a thousand women man; I invoke the waters, plants, animals, the earth, the fire, the sun, the air and the whole of nature; I invoke all the chemical elements that make up my sacred body; I invoke the spirits of justice to demonstrate your power, 'that my body overflowing vigor, health and mood for love; that is able to meet many women, until the last days of my life '. My glance a woman do my veins dilate, my penis harden like rock firm and my whole body is ready to satisfy them, is when, with whom and for me to come will, respecting the privacy of my brothers and sisters. In gratitude what I'm getting, I promise to be a gentleman, fair, polite, loving, charitable and diligent with all my fellow men and women I have come to this as lovers, now and ever and ever. "

Every day, before dinner, take 1/4 cup of the wine above.

DO NOT PASS BY THIS SITE, for SEVEN MONTHS.

15 - Sword

Materials

1 kit enthroned spells

12 "swords-of-are-jorge";

12 cloves of whole garlic and raw;

01 white cloth of 0.60 m x 1 m;

Strings or masking tape;

07 filled branches of rosemary;

01 shirt or red shirt, virgin, entirely;

12 ginger slices 2 cm in length (more or less).

Preparation

One evening crescent, put the ingredients on the kit spells;

Join the swords, ginger and garlic cloves;

Wrap them properly in white cloth;

Pass masking tape, or string, the middle and the ends;

Put this package in the moonlight, for 12 minutes;

Place the rosemary sprigs in a container with 02 liters of water and boil for five minutes;

Let cool and bathe with this liquid, not dry;

Place this package under the bed, you go to sleep - in the longitudinal direction, ie the length of the bed - by lying next;

Store the kit and other items.

Dispatch

The next morning, given the shirt or shirt, red skirt and with this package;

Let this package, against a Christian church.

Prayer

Made the order, take twelve steps forward, not looking back, and recite, with great faith and steadfastness the following prayer:

"Al-ilah Rapha, very precious and exalted Lord who Heals, examines my body and my physical nature with Thy penetrating Healing Power. That Thou me Cures of all diseases and sufferings and bring me the restoration of body and spirit for me that I now pray and especially for those who are going through a transition process".

XXXXXXXXXXXX